Gallbladder diet cookbook 2024

Revitalize Your Metabolism with Flavorful and Nourishing Recipes

Viukuthla zoaka

COPYRIGHT PAGE

TABLE OF CONTENTS

CHAPTER 4 SNACKING SMART FOR GALLBLADDER WELLNESS........................54

CHAPTER 5 FLAVORFUL DINNERS THAT SUPPORT GALLBLADDER FUNCTION.............64

CHAPTER 1
UNDERSTANDING THE GALLBLADDER DIET

An Introduction to the Gallbladder Diet

The gallbladder is a tiny organ located under the liver that plays an important function in digestion. It helps to store and release bile, which is necessary for the breakdown of lipids during digestion. While the gallbladder is sometimes disregarded, its importance becomes clear when problems emerge, resulting in digestive pain and disturbances. The gallbladder diet is a starting point for understanding the dietary changes required to keep the gallbladder healthy and avoid issues.

The gallbladder diet focuses on improving nutrition to maintain gallbladder function and lowering the risk of gallbladder-related issues. Whether you've had gallbladder problems in the past or are looking for strategies to improve digestive health, eating a gallbladder-friendly diet can help you feel better overall.

In this complete examination of the gallbladder diet, we will look at the necessity of a healthy gallbladder, frequent concerns that may emerge, the basic rules regulating this specialized diet, and a full guide to items that should be consumed or avoided. Individuals who understand these characteristics may make educated decisions to promote gallbladder health while still enjoying a balanced and nutritious diet.

The importance of a healthy gallbladder

The gallbladder stores bile, a digestive fluid generated by the liver. This bile is discharged into the small intestine to help in the digestion of dietary lipids. A healthy gallbladder promotes effective digestion and nutrition absorption, playing an important role in overall digestive health.

1. *Digestion Efficiency:*
A healthy gallbladder ensures that bile is discharged at the proper times. This enables for efficient fat emulsification, which facilitates enzyme digestion and aids in the absorption of important fatty acids and fat soluble vitamins.

2. *Preventing gallstones:*

The production of gallstones is one of the most common gallbladder issues. These solid particles can form when the chemicals in bile become imbalanced, resulting in crystallization. A healthy gallbladder has a lower risk of developing gallstones, which can cause discomfort, inflammation, and other issues.

3. *Regulation of Cholesterol Levels*

The gallbladder helps to keep the body's cholesterol levels balanced. Proper management inhibits the buildup of excess cholesterol in the bile, lowering the risk of gallstone development and boosting cardiovascular health.

4. *Optimized Nutrient Absorption:*

The gallbladder indirectly aids in fat digestion, which aids in the absorption of fat-soluble vitamins A, D, E, and K. These vitamins are required for a variety of body processes, including immune system support, bone health, and eyesight.

5. Improved Digestive Comfort: A healthy gallbladder leads to better digestion, decreasing pain, bloating, and other signs of poor bile flow.

An Overview of Common Gallbladder Issues

Gallbladder problems can take many forms, ranging from minor concerns to more serious disorders that necessitate medical intervention. Being aware of these concerns allows people to notice possible signs and take preventative measures to resolve them. Here's a summary of some typical gallbladder issues:

1. *Gallstones:*

Gallstones are solid particles that develop within the gallbladder. They vary in size and can cause pain and discomfort if they obstruct the passage of bile. Symptoms of gallstones include stomach discomfort, nausea, vomiting, and inflammation.

2. Cholecystitis:*

Cholecystitis is an inflammation of the gallbladder caused by gallstones that clog the bile ducts. Acute cholecystitis can cause significant discomfort, fever, and consequences if not treated soon.

3. *Biliary Dyskinesia*

Biliary dyskinesia is a condition defined by decreased gallbladder function. The gallbladder may not contract and discharge bile properly, resulting in symptoms such as discomfort, indigestion, and nausea.

4. *Gallbladder polyps:*

Polyps are growths that can form on the inside lining of the gallbladder. While most gallbladder polyps are benign, some may need to be monitored or removed if they have the potential to become malignant.

5. *Gallbladder Cancer*

Gallbladder cancer is possible, however rare. It frequently manifests with vague symptoms, making early identification difficult. Age, gender, and certain medical conditions all contribute to the risk of gallbladder cancer.

Important Principles of the Gallbladder Diet

The gallbladder diet is based on three principles: promote digestive health, reduce the risk of gallbladder problems, and ensure adequate nutritional absorption. These important ideas help people make dietary decisions that promote gallbladder function. Here are the basic concepts of the gallbladder diet:

1. Moderation of Dietary Fats:*
   While fats are necessary for general health, they must be consumed in moderation to ensure gallbladder health. Excessive consumption of high-fat meals might cause the release of more bile, potentially leading to gallbladder pain and symptoms. Limit your intake of saturated and trans fats and instead go for healthy fats like olive oil, almonds, and avocado.

2. Emphasis on Fiber-Rich Foods:

A fiber-rich diet improves intestinal health and helps to manage cholesterol levels. Fruits, vegetables, whole grains, and legumes are all high-fiber foods that can help avoid gallstones and promote regular bowel movements.

3. *Adequate Hydration*
Staying hydrated is vital for maintaining biliary fluidity. Drinking enough of water helps to keep bile from concentrating, lowering the chance of gallstones. It also promotes overall digestive function and general well-being.

4. Lean Protein Sources: Eating chicken, fish, and plant-based proteins can improve gallbladder health. These proteins digest more easily and do not irritate the gallbladder as much as high-fat meats.

5. Balanced Meals and Regular Eating Patterns:

Adopting a regular, balanced food plan promotes gallbladder function. Skipping meals or following irregular eating habits might result in concentrated bile, increasing the risk of gallstone development.

6. Mindful Eating Practices:*
Mindful eating entails paying attention to hunger and fullness signs, chewing deeply, and relishing every meal. This exercise improves healthy digestion and helps to avoid overeating, which can strain the gallbladder.

7. Limitation of Trigger Foods:
Some people may discover that particular meals cause gallbladder issues. These can include spicy, oily, or fried meals, as well as dairy products. Identifying and restricting the use of trigger foods can help

Gallbladder comfort.

8. *Inclusion of Gallbladder Supportive Herbs:*
   Certain herbs and spices have been traditionally linked to gallbladder health. Herbs that may help with digestion include turmeric, ginger, peppermint, and dandelion. Including them in recipes or drinks might be a tasty approach to promote gallbladder function.

9. *How to Maintain a Healthy Body Weight:*
   Obesity has long been associated with gallbladder problems, particularly the production of gallstones. Maintaining a healthy body weight with a balanced diet and frequent physical activity might improve gallbladder health.

10. *Individualized Approach*
   Recognizing that everyone's nutritional demands and tolerances are different, the gallbladder diet promotes a personalized

approach. What works for one person may not work for another, and changes may be required depending on personal tastes, medical problems, and reactions to certain foods.

Adhering to these fundamental guidelines establishes the foundation for a gallbladder-friendly lifestyle. Individual reactions to meals might vary, so speaking with a healthcare practitioner or a certified dietitian can provide individualized advice for people with unique gallbladder difficulties.

Foods to Enjoy and Avoid

Making conscious eating selections is essential while following the gallbladder diet. Certain foods are considered favorable to gallbladder health, while others should be taken in moderation or avoided. Understanding these characteristics enables people to choose a diet that promotes gallbladder function. Here's a full list of foods to embrace and avoid when following the gallbladder diet:

Foods to embrace:

1. Eat a range of colored fruits and vegetables, including apples, pears, berries, kale, spinach, and broccoli. These foods are high in fiber, vitamins, and antioxidants.

2. Choose whole grains, like quinoa, brown rice, oats, and whole wheat. These grains provide fiber and aid with digestive health.

3. Choose lean protein sources, such as poultry, fish, tofu, lentils, and plant-based protein. These solutions are gentler on the digestive tract and do not overwork the gallbladder.

4. *Healthy Fats:* Incorporate healthy fats like avocados, nuts, seeds, and olive oil. These fats promote general health while putting less load on the gallbladder.

5. *Low-Fat Dairy and Alternatives:*
   - Choose low-fat or fat-free dairy products, or dairy substitutes such as almond or soymilk. These solutions supply critical nutrients without the high fat level of full-fat dairy.

6. Use herbs and spices such as turmeric, ginger, peppermint, and dandelion in cooking. These herbs have long been connected with digestive benefits and can provide taste without causing gallbladder pain.

7. Stay hydrated by drinking plenty of water throughout the day. Hydration increases bile fluidity and improves overall digestive function.

8. Consume fiber-rich foods, including beans, lentils, whole grains, fruits, and vegetables. Fiber promotes digestion and regulates cholesterol levels.

9. Moderate Consumption of Healthy Oils:
   - Use healthy oils, such as olive oil, in moderation. These oils supply vital fatty acids without overpowering the gallbladder.

10. Eat probiotic-rich foods including yogurt, kefir, sauerkraut, and kimchi. These foods promote gut health, which is associated with general digestive well-being.

Foods to avoid or limit

1. Foods with high fat content: Limit your consumption of high-fat meals, such as fried dishes, fatty cuts of meat, and processed snacks. Excessive fat consumption can stimulate the gallbladder, causing pain.

2. *Spicy meals:* Some people may get gallbladder symptoms after eating spicy meals. Monitor your own tolerance and consider reducing or avoiding spicy foods.

3. Reduce intake of processed and packaged foods, as they typically include chemicals, preservatives, and harmful fats that might affect gallbladder health.

4. Limit full-fat dairy intake to reduce bile concentration and risk of gallstone development.

5. *Red Meat:* - Consume moderate amounts of red meat, particularly fatty slices. Choose leaner protein sources, such as poultry and fish.

6. *Excessive Caffeine:* - Moderate caffeine intake is normally okay, but excessive use may lead to gallbladder difficulties.

CHAPTER 2 NOURISHING BREAKFASTS FOR GALLBLADDER HEALTH

Avocado and Egg Breakfast Bowl

Ingredients:

- One ripe avocado.

- Two poached eggs

- Halved cherry tomatoes - Optional garnish with chia seeds

Instructions:

1. Cut a ripe avocado in half and remove the pit.

2. Scoop out some of the avocado to make a well for the eggs.

3. Poach the eggs to your preference.

4. Place a poached egg in each avocado half.

5. Optionally, garnish with halved cherry tomatoes and chia seeds.

6. Add salt and pepper to taste.

7. Savor your Avocado and Egg Breakfast Bowl!

Berry-Almond Smoothie

Ingredients:

Ingredients: 1 cup mixed berries (blueberries, raspberries), 1 cup almond milk, and 1 scoop protein powder.

- A handful of chopped almonds.

Instructions:

1. In a blender, combine the mixed berries, almond milk, and protein powder.

2. Blend until smooth and creamy.

3. Pour the smoothie into a glass.

4. Garnish with chopped almonds.

5. Add the almonds to the smoothie or enjoy as a crunchy topping.

6. Serve and enjoy your Berry and Almond Smoothie

Chia Seed Pudding with Mango

Ingredients:

- Two teaspoons of chia seeds

Ingredients: 1 cup almond milk, 1 diced mango, and a drizzle of honey.

Instructions:

1. In a dish, combine chia seeds and almond milk.

2. Mix thoroughly and refrigerate overnight or for at least 4 hours, until the liquid thickens.

3. In a serving glass or dish, combine the chia pudding and chopped mango.

4. Drizzle honey on top.

5. Gently mix before eating to incorporate all of the flavors.

6. Enjoy the Chia Seed Pudding with Mango!

Greek yogurt parfait

Ingredients:

- Greek Yogurt

Ingredients: granola, fresh strawberries (sliced), and flaxseeds

Instructions:

1. In a glass or dish, layer the Greek yogurt.

2. Sprinkle granola on top of the yogurt.

3. Top the granola with cut strawberries.

4. Repeat the layers until the glass is full.

5. Finish with a sprinkling of flaxseed.

6. Serve and enjoy your healthful Greek Yogurt Parfait!

Spinach and Feta Omelette

Ingredients

- Eggs

- Fresh spinach, chopped.

- Feta cheese crumbled

- Cherry tomatoes halved

- Add salt and pepper to taste.

Instructions:

1. In a bowl, whisk together the eggs and season with salt and pepper.

2. In a skillet, cook the chopped spinach until wilted.

3. Pour the whisked eggs over the spinach.

4. Spread crumbled feta and halved cherry tomatoes over one side of the omelet.

5. Fold the omelet over the filling, then cook until the eggs are set.

6. Transfer the omelet to a platter.

7. Optionally, garnish with more feta and cherry tomatoes.

8. Serve the Spinach and Feta Omelet hot.

Quinoa Breakfast Bowl

Ingredients:

Ingredients include cooked quinoa with sliced banana.

Ingredients include chopped walnuts and maple syrup.

Instructions:

1. In a bowl, combine cooked quinoa and sliced banana.

2. Toss chopped walnuts into the quinoa and banana mixture.

3. Drizzle with maple syrup for extra richness.

4. Combine thoroughly and enjoy your nutritious Quinoa Breakfast Bowl!

Oatmeal With Berries And Almond Butter

Ingredients

Ingredients include rolled oats, mixed berries, and almond butter.

- Cinnamon

Instructions:

1. Cook the rolled oats according per the package directions.

2. Sprinkle the oats with mixed berries.

3. Add a dab of almond butter.

4. Sprinkle cinnamon on top.

5. Combine the ingredients before eating your Oatmeal with Berries and Almond Butter!

Buckwheat Pancakes With Fresh Berries

Ingredients:

- Buckwheat flour - Almond milk.

- Eggs - Fresh Berries

- Maple syrup.

Instructions:

1. In a bowl, combine the buckwheat flour, almond milk, and eggs to make pancake batter.

2. Make pancakes on a griddle or in a pan.

3. Top with fresh berries.

4. Drizzle with maple syrup.

5. Serve warm and enjoy your Buckwheat Pancakes with Fresh Berries!

Vegetable and Herbal Frittata

Ingredients

- Eggs

- Bell peppers, diced

Zucchini (sliced)

- Cherry tomatoes halved

- Fresh herbs (parsley, chives)

- Add salt and pepper to taste.

Instructions

1. In a bowl, whisk together the eggs and season with salt and pepper.

2. Cook chopped bell peppers, zucchini, and cherry tomatoes in an oven-safe pan.

3. Pour the whisked eggs over the veggies.

4. Sprinkle some fresh herbs on top.

5. Bake in the oven until the frittata has set.

6. Let it cool slightly before slicing and serving the Veggie and Herb Frittata.

Coconut Chia Seed Smoothie Bowl

Ingredients

- Coconut milk - ChIa seeds, sliced kiwi, and shredded coconut.

Instructions

1. Combine coconut milk and chia seeds.

2. Refrigerate for at least 4 hours or overnight to thicken the mixture.

3. Transfer the chia seed mixture to a bowl.

4. Garnish with sliced kiwi and shredded coconut.

5. Gently mix before eating to blend tastes.

6. Savor your delightful Coconut Chia Seed Smoothie Bowl!

CHAPTER 3
WHOLESOME LUNCHES TO SUPPORT YOUR GALLBLADDER

Grilled Chicken and Vegetable Wraps

Ingredients

- Grilled chicken breast slices.

- Colorful veggies (cherry tomatoes, bell peppers, and zucchini).

- Whole grain tortillas.

- Olive Oil

- Fresh herbs (like basil and cilantro)

- Add salt and pepper to taste.

Instructions

1. Season the chicken breast pieces with salt and pepper, then sprinkle with olive oil.

2. Grill the chicken until it is well cooked and slightly browned.

3. In a separate skillet, sauté the colorful veggies until soft and crisp.

4. Warm the whole grain tortillas.

5. Make the wraps by arranging grilled chicken slices and sautéed veggies in the middle of each tortilla.

6. Add fresh herbs to the fillings.

7. Fold the tortilla's edges over the ingredients, then roll to form a wrap.

8. Secure with toothpicks if necessary.

9. Serve the grilled chicken and vegetable wraps warm.

Quinoa and Chickpea Salad

Ingredients

- Cooked quinoa - Canned chickpeas (drained and rinsed).

- Cucumber diced

- Cherry tomatoes halved

- Fresh herbs, like parsley or mint.

- Lemon Vinaigrette (lemon juice, olive oil, Dijon mustard, salt, and pepper)

Instructions

1. In a large mixing bowl, add cooked quinoa, chickpeas, chopped cucumber, and split cherry tomatoes.

2. For added taste, stir in chopped fresh herbs.

3. In a small dish, combine the lemon vinaigrette ingredients.

4. Pour the vinaigrette over the salad and gently toss to mix.

5. Refrigerate for at least 30 minutes to let the flavors combine.

6. Serve the Quinoa and Chickpea Salad cold.

Tasty Lentil Soups & Stews

Ingredients

- Dried lentils.

- Vegetables (carrots, celery, and onions).

- Garlic, minced

- Vegetable or chicken broth - Herbs and spices (e.g., thyme, bay leaves, cumin).

- Add salt and pepper to taste.

Instructions

1. Rinse and drain the dried lentils.

2. In a large saucepan, cook the minced garlic, onions, carrots, and celery until tender.

3. Put the lentils, broth, thyme, bay leaves, and cumin into the pot.

4. Bring to a boil, then decrease the heat and simmer until the lentils are cooked.

5. Add salt and pepper to taste.

6. Remove the bay leaves before serving.

7. Serve the Satisfying Lentil Soup in bowls and enjoy.

Baked Fish With Citrus Infusions

Ingredients

- Fish filets (tilapia or cod).

- Citrus fruits (lime or lemon), sliced

- Fresh herbs (like parsley or dill).

- Olive Oil

- Add salt and pepper to taste.

Instructions

1. Preheat your oven to 375°F (190°C).

2. Transfer the fish filets to a baking dish.

3. Drizzle olive oil over the fish, then season with salt and pepper.

4. Place citrus slices and fresh herbs on top of the fish.

5. Bake in the preheated oven for 15-20 minutes, or until the fish is thoroughly cooked and readily flaked.

6. Prior to serving, garnish with more fresh herbs.

7. Serve the baked fish with citrus infusions among steamed veggies or quinoa.

Veggie-Packed Buddha Bowls

Ingredients

- Roasted or sautéed veggies (such as sweet potatoes, broccoli, and kale).

- cooked quinoa or brown rice.

- Avocado slices.

- Canned chickpeas (drained and washed)

- Tahini Dressing

Instructions

1. Roast or sauté the veggies until they're soft.

2. Fill the Buddha bowls with quinoa or brown rice, one serving per bowl.

3. Combine the roasted or sautéed veggies, avocado slices, and chickpeas.

4. Drizzle with tahini dressing to add flavor.

5. Toss lightly to blend, or keep the ingredients separate for a visually pleasing presentation.

6. Serve the Veggie-Packed Buddha Bowls warm or room temperature.

Grilled Salmon and Lemon Dill Sauce

Ingredients

- Salmon Filets
- Make lemon dill sauce using mayonnaise or Greek yogurt, lemon juice, fresh dill, salt, and pepper. - Use olive oil.
- Add salt and pepper to taste.

Instructions

1. Preheat the grill to medium-high.
2. Coat the salmon filets in olive oil and season with salt and pepper.
3. Grill the salmon for 4-5 minutes on each side, or until it achieves the desired doneness.
4. In a small dish, combine the lemon dill sauce ingredients.
5. Just before serving, spoon the sauce over the cooked fish.

6. If preferred, garnish with more fresh dill.

7. Serve the Grilled Salmon with Lemon Dill Sauce alongside steamed asparagus or green beans.

Roasted Turkey Breast and Herbed Quinoa

Ingredients

- Roasted turkey breast slices

- Herbed quinoa (quinoa, vegetable or chicken broth, fresh herbs) - Sautéed Brussels sprouts or green veggies

- Olive Oil

- Add salt and pepper to taste.

Instructions

1. Roast or grill turkey breast pieces until well done.

2. To make herbed quinoa, simmer the quinoa in broth and add fresh herbs.

3. Sauté Brussels sprouts or other green veggies in olive oil until they're soft.

4. To assemble the meal, place turkey slices over a bed of herbed quinoa with sautéed veggies on the side.

5. Add salt and pepper to taste.

6. Pair the Roasted Turkey Breast with Herbed Quinoa for a filling and healthful meal.

Vegetable stir-fry with tofu

Ingredients

- Tofu cubed

- Mixed veggies (e.g. broccoli, bell peppers, snap peas, carrots) - Minced ginger

- Garlic, minced

- Low sodium soy sauce

Sesame oil

- Brown rice, quinoa

Instructions

1. Cook the cubed tofu in sesame oil until golden brown.

2. Add minced ginger and garlic to the pan and cook for 1-2 minutes.

3. Add the veggies and continue to stir-fry until soft and crispy.

4. Pour the low-sodium soy sauce over the tofu and veggies.

5. Serve the veggie stir-fry over cooked brown rice or quinoa.

6. If desired, garnish with more sesame oil or seeds.

7. Enjoy the Vegetable Stir-Fry with Tofu for a wonderful and nutritious meal.

Spaghetti squash primavera

Ingredients

- Spaghetti squash - Mixed veggies (cherry tomatoes, spinach, mushrooms) - Olive oil.

- Garlic, minced

- Pesto or tomato sauce.

 Chop fresh basil and season with salt and pepper to taste.

Instructions

1. Preheat your oven to 375°F (190°C).

2. Cut the spaghetti squash in half lengthwise, remove the seeds, and lay on a baking pan.

3. Roast the spaghetti squash in the oven for 40–45 minutes, or until the flesh is soft.

4. While the squash roasts, sauté various veggies and chopped garlic in olive oil until done.

5. With a fork, scrape the cooked spaghetti squash into strands.

6. Combine the spaghetti squash strands with the sautéed veggies and a choice of tomato sauce or pesto.

7. Add salt and pepper to taste.

8. Just before serving, garnish with freshly chopped basil.

9. Serve Spaghetti Squash Primavera as a lighter option to conventional pasta recipes.

Comforting Lentil and Brown Rice Casserole

Ingredients

Cooked brown rice and lentils.

- Mixed veggies (carrots, peas, and corn).

- Tomato sauce or vegetable broth - Herbs and spices (e.g., oregano, thyme, garlic powder).

- grated cheese (optional).

- Add salt and pepper to taste.

Instructions

1. Preheat your oven to 375°F (190°C).

2. In a large mixing bowl, add the cooked brown rice, lentils, mixed vegetables, tomato sauce or vegetable broth, and herbs and spices.

3. Add salt and pepper to taste.

4. Place the mixture in a baking dish.

5. If desired, add shredded cheese on top.

6. Bake in the preheated oven for 20-25 minutes, or until the casserole is fully cooked and the top is golden brown.

7. Allow it to cool somewhat before serving.

8. Serve the Comforting Lentil and Brown Rice Casserole for a nutritious and filling meal.

CHAPTER 4 SNACKING SMART FOR GALLBLADDER WELLNESS

Fresh fruit slices with almond butter

Ingredients

- Sliced fruits (apples, pears, or bananas) - Almond butter

Instructions

1. Wash and cut the appropriate fruit into bite-size pieces.

2. Place the fruit slices on a platter.

3. Transfer almond butter to a small bowl or immediately onto a plate.

4. Before eating the fruit pieces, dip or spread them with almond butter.

Greek Yogurt Parfait

Ingredients

- Low-fat Greek yogurt.

- Fresh fruits (strawberries, blueberries, raspberries) - Granola - Honey

Instructions

1. In a glass or dish, layer Greek yogurt on the bottom.

2. Arrange a layer of fresh berries on top of the yogurt.

3. Sprinkle granola over the berries.

4. Repeat the layers until the container is full.

5. Drizzle honey over top for sweetness.

6. Use a large spoon to eat the layers individually or combine them for a delicious parfait experience.

Roasted Chickpeas

Ingredients

- Drain and rinse canned chickpeas - Add olive oil, cumin, paprika, and salt.

Instructions

1. Preheat your oven to 400°F (200°C).
2. Dry the chickpeas with a paper towel.
3. In a bowl, combine the chickpeas, olive oil, cumin, paprika, and salt to taste.
4. Arrange the chickpeas in a single layer on a baking sheet.

5. Roast in the preheated oven for 25-30 minutes or until crispy, stirring the pan regularly to ensure equal cooking.

6. Let the roasted chickpeas cool before serving.

Rice Cake and Avocado

Ingredients

- Brown Rice Cakes

- Ripe avocados.

Ingredients include sea salt and lemon juice.

Instructions

1. Cut the avocado in half, remove the pit, and scoop out the flesh into a dish.

2. Using a fork, mash the avocado and squeeze in some lemon juice.

3. Spread the mashed avocado on the rice cakes.

4. Add a pinch of sea salt on top.

5. Serve immediately as a simple and filling snack.

Veggie Sticks and Hummus

Ingredients

Carrot sticks, cucumber sticks, and hummus

Instructions

1. Wash carrots and cucumbers, then cut them into stick shapes.
2. Arrange the vegetable sticks on a platter.
3. Serve with a side of hummus to dip.

Cottage Cheese and Pineapple Cups

Ingredients

- Use low-fat cottage cheese and fresh pineapple chunks.

Instructions

1. Spoon one serving of low-fat cottage cheese into a dish or cup.

2. Top the cottage cheese with fresh pineapple pieces.

3. Savor the mix of creamy cottage cheese and juicy pineapple.

Trail Mix With Nuts And Dried Fruit

Ingredients

Almonds, walnuts, dried apricots, and raisins.

Instructions

1. Measure out the required amount of almonds, walnuts, dried apricots, and raisins.

2. Combine the items in a bowl.

3. Divide the trail mix into tiny snack-sized bags for convenient, on-the-go consumption.

Whole Grain Crackers and Smoked Salmon

Ingredients

Ingredients: Whole grain crackers with smoked salmon.

- Lemon wedges.

Instructions

1. Arrange the whole grain crackers on a dish.

2. Arrange thin slices of smoked salmon on top of each cracker.

3. Garnish with lemon wedges for an extra punch of citrus.

Hard Boiled Eggs

Ingredients

- Eggs - Season with salt and pepper to taste.

Instructions

1. Put the eggs in a pot and cover with water.
2. Bring the water to a boil, then decrease heat and simmer for 10 minutes.
3. Remove the eggs from the boiling water and allow them to cool.
4. Peel the eggs and season with salt and pepper before eating.

Berry and Cottage Cheese Bowl

Ingredients

- Low-fat cottage cheese - Mixed berries (strawberries, blueberries, and raspberries)

Instructions

1. In a bowl, place a serving of low-fat cottage cheese.

2. Top the cottage cheese with a mixture of berries.

3. Gently fold the berries into the cottage cheese, or serve them stacked.

CHAPTER 5 FLAVORFUL DINNERS THAT SUPPORT GALLBLADDER FUNCTION

Grilled Chicken and Lemon-Herb Quinoa

Ingredients

Ingredients include chicken breast and lemon.

- Fresh herbs (parsley, thyme, or rosemary).

Ingredients include quinoa and olive oil.

Add salt and pepper to taste. Serve over steamed green beans.

Instructions

1. To marinate the chicken breast, combine olive oil, lemon juice, chopped fresh herbs, salt, and pepper.

2. Grill the chicken until thoroughly done, with a beautiful brown on the edges.

3. Meanwhile, prepare the quinoa according to package directions, adding a squeeze of lemon juice and chopped herbs.

4. Serve the grilled chicken over lemon-herb quinoa, with steamed green beans on the side.

Baked Salmon With Dill And Asparagus

Ingredients

Ingredients include salmon filets, fresh dill, and lemon.

Ingredients include asparagus spears and olive oil.

- Add salt and pepper to taste.

- Quinoa or brown rice (optional for serving).

Instructions

1. Preheat your oven to 375°F (190°C).

2. Transfer the salmon filets to a baking sheet.

3. Sprinkle the salmon with chopped fresh dill, lemon slices, olive oil, salt, and pepper.

4. Arrange the asparagus spears around the salmon.

5. Bake in the preheated oven for 15-20 minutes, or until the salmon is well cooked.

6. Optionally, serve the baked salmon and asparagus over quinoa or brown rice.

Lentils and Vegetable Curry

Ingredients

- Dry lentils - Mixed veggies (such as carrots, bell peppers, peas)

- Coconut Milk

- Curry spices: turmeric, cumin, and coriander

- Onion

- Garlic

- Ginger - Olive oil.

- Basmati rice (to serve)

Instructions

1. Rinse and drain the lentils.

2. In a saucepan, sauté chopped onion, garlic, and ginger in olive oil until aromatic.

3. Add the curry spices and stir.

4. Add the mixed veggies and lentils to the pot.

5. Pour in the coconut milk and allow it to boil until the lentils and veggies are cooked.

6. Serve the lentil and vegetable stew over basmati rice.

Stir-Fry with Turkey and Vegetables

Ingredients

- Use lean ground turkey, mixed veggies (broccoli, bell peppers, snap peas), and low-sodium soy sauce.

- Ginger - Garlic.

- Olive Oil

- Brown rice or quinoa (to serve)

Instructions

1. In a wok or big skillet, cook the ground turkey in olive oil until browned.

2. Add minced ginger and garlic to the pan and cook for 1-2 minutes.

3. Add the mixed veggies and continue to stir-fry until cooked and crisp.

4. Pour the low-sodium soy sauce over the turkey and veggies.

5. Serve the turkey and veggie stir-fry over brown rice or quinoa.

Quinoa-stuffed Bell Peppers

Ingredients

Bell peppers, quinoa, black beans, corn, and diced tomatoes.

Ingredients: - Cumin - Chili Powder

Optional toppings include olive oil and low-fat cheese.

Instructions

1. Preheat your oven to 375°F (190°C).

2. Cut bell peppers in half and remove the seeds and membranes.

3. Cook the quinoa according to the package directions.

4. In a bowl, combine cooked quinoa, black beans, corn, diced tomatoes, cumin, chili powder, and a sprinkle of olive oil.

5. Fill each bell pepper half with quinoa mixture.

6. Optionally, top with low-fat cheese.

7. Bake in a preheated oven for 20-25 minutes,
or until the peppers are soft.

Shrimp and vegetable skewers

Ingredients

Ingredients include peeled and deveined shrimp
and cherry tomatoes.

Zucchini, sliced

Cut bell peppers into pieces and drizzle with
olive oil.

- Garlic

- Lemon Juice

- Fresh parsley for garnish.

- Couscous (to serve)

Instructions

1. In a bowl, toss shrimp, cherry tomatoes, zucchini, and bell peppers with olive oil, garlic, and lemon juice.

2. Thread the marinated items on skewers.

3. Grill the skewers until the shrimp is fully cooked and the veggies are browned.

4. Serve the shrimp and vegetable skewers on a bed of couscous, topped with fresh parsley.

Herb-Roasted Chicken Thighs with Sweet Potatoes

Ingredients

- Chicken thighs.

- Peeled and diced sweet potatoes - Fresh herbs (e.g., rosemary, thyme)

- Olive Oil

- Garlic

- Season with salt and pepper to taste. - Serve over steamed broccoli.

Instructions

1. Preheat your oven to 400°F (200°C).
2. In a mixing dish, combine chicken thighs and diced sweet potatoes with olive oil, chopped garlic, fresh herbs, salt, and pepper.
3. Place the chicken and sweet potatoes on a baking pan.
4. Roast in the preheated oven for 30-35 minutes, or until the chicken is thoroughly cooked and the sweet potatoes are soft.
5. Serve the herb-roasted chicken thighs with steamed broccoli as a side.

Spinach-Mushroom Quiche

Ingredients

- Whole grain pie crust - Eggs - Low-fat milk or milk substitute

Ingredients include fresh spinach, sliced mushrooms, diced onion, and low-fat cheese.

- Add salt and pepper to taste.

Instructions

1. Preheat your oven to 375°F (190°C).

2. In a pan, sauté the chopped onion, sliced mushrooms, and fresh spinach until softened.

3. In a bowl, combine the eggs, low-fat milk, salt, and pepper.

4. Put the whole-grain pie dough into a pie plate.

5. Spread the sautéed veggies over the crust, then pour the egg mixture over them.

6. Top with low-fat cheese.

7. Bake the quiche in the preheated oven for 30-35 minutes, or until set and golden brown.

Zucchini Noodles With Pesto And Grilled Chicken

Ingredients

- Zucchini with grilled chicken breast.

Ingredients: - Basil pesto - Halved cherry tomatoes

- Pine nuts (optional as garnish)

- Parmesan cheese (optional; for topping)

Instructions

1. Use a spiralizer to make zucchini noodles (zoodles).

2. Grill chicken breast until thoroughly done, then slice into strips.

3. In a pan, cook zucchini noodles until barely soft.

4. Combine the zoodles with the basil pesto, grilled chicken strips, and halved cherry tomatoes.

5. Before serving, garnish with pine nuts and sprinkle with Parmesan cheese.

Baked cod with tomato and olive relish

Ingredients

Ingredients: cod filets, chopped cherry tomatoes, and kalam

Sliced ata olives, finely chopped red onion, chopped fresh parsley, olive oil, and lemon juice.

Add salt and pepper to taste. Serve over quinoa or wild rice.

Instructions

1. Preheat your oven to 375°F (190°C).

2. Season the cod filets with olive oil, lemon juice, salt, and pepper.

3. Transfer the fish filets to a baking sheet.

4. In a bowl, combine diced cherry tomatoes, sliced Kalamata olives, finely chopped red onion, and fresh parsley.

5. Spread the tomato and olive relish on the fish filets.

6. Bake in the preheated oven for 15-20 minutes, or until the fish is well cooked.

7. Serve the roasted fish with tomato and olive relish over quinoa or wild rice.

CHAPTER 6 DESSERTS AND TREATS

Apple Cinnamon Baked Oatmeal

Ingredients

- 2 cups rolled oats - 1 teaspoon baking powder.

- One teaspoon of ground cinnamon

- 1/4 teaspoon salt - 2 cups milk (dairy or vegan)

- 1/4 cup maple syrup.

Ingredients: 2 peeled and sliced apples, 1/2 cup chopped nuts (optional).

Ingredients: 1 tablespoon melted butter or coconut oil, 1 teaspoon vanilla essence.

Instructions

1. Preheat the oven to 350°F/175°C and butter a baking dish.

2. In a bowl, mix the oats, baking powder, cinnamon, and salt.

3. In another dish, combine the milk, maple syrup, melted butter or coconut oil, and vanilla extract.

4. Pour the wet components over the dry ingredients, stirring to incorporate.

5. Gently fold in the chopped apples and nuts.

6. Pour the mixture into the prepared baking dish.

7. Bake for 30–35 minutes, or until the top is brown and the oatmeal has set.

8. Allow it to cool somewhat before serving.

Banana and Almond Butter Bites

Ingredients

Bananas, sliced

- Almond Butter

- Chia seeds are optional.

- Sliced almonds are optional.

Instructions

1. Cut the bananas into bite-sized pieces.

2. Spread a little quantity of almond butter onto each banana slice.

3. Optional: Add chia seeds or sliced almonds for texture.

4. Place the banana and almond butter bits on a tray.

5. Serve immediately for a fast and nutritious snack.

Chia Seed Pudding with Berries

Ingredients

- 1/4 cup chia seeds.

- Add 1 cup almond milk and 1 tablespoon honey or maple syrup.

- Mixed berries, including strawberries, blueberries, and raspberries.

Instructions

1. In a jar or dish, combine the chia seeds, almond milk, and honey/maple syrup.

2. Stir thoroughly to remove any clumps, then refrigerate for at least 2 hours or overnight.

3. Just before serving, mix the chia pudding again.

4. Pour the chia pudding into serving glasses or bowls and top with mixed berries.

5. Sprinkle with extra berries on top.

Dark Chocolate Dipped Strawberries

Ingredients

- Wash and dry fresh strawberries. - Melt dark chocolate.

Instructions

1. Melt the dark chocolate in a heatproof basin.
2. Dip each strawberry in the melted chocolate, covering halfway or as desired.
3. Arrange the chocolate-dipped strawberries on a parchment-lined dish.
4. Let the chocolate set in the refrigerator for 15-20 minutes.
5. Serve chilled and enjoy these lovely yet easy delights.

Greek Yogurt Parfait With Nuts and Honey

Ingredients

- Low-fat Greek yogurt.

Chop mixed nuts (almonds, walnuts) and add honey.

Instructions

1. In a glass or dish, arrange low-fat Greek yogurt.

2. Sprinkle the chopped nuts over the yogurt.

3. Drizzle honey over the top for sweetness.

4. Repeat the layers as required.

5. Serve immediately for a protein-rich and fulfilling parfait.

Honey-Sweetened Fruit Salad

Ingredients

- Fresh fruits (including berries, melons, grapes, and citrus) - Honey

Instructions

1. Wash, peel, and cut the fresh fruit into bite-sized pieces.

2. Mix the fruits in a basin.

3. Drizzle honey over the fruit salad and gently mix to combine.

4. Refrigerate for at least 30 minutes before serving to let the flavors combine.

Coconut and Berries Ice Pops

Ingredients

- Coconut water - Mixed berries (strawberries, blueberries, and raspberries)

Instructions

1. Fill ice pop molds with mixed berries.

2. Pour coconut water over the fruit until the molds are filled.

3. Insert the ice pop sticks and freeze for at least four hours, or until solid.

4. Run the molds under warm water to remove the popsicles.

5. Indulge in these delightful and nourishing coconut and berry ice pops.

Baked Apples With Cinnamon And Walnuts

Ingredients

- Cored and halved apples - Ground cinnamon - Chopped walnuts.

- Honey

Instructions

1. Preheat your oven to 375°F (190°C).

2. Arrange the cored and halved apples on a baking sheet.

3. Sprinkle ground cinnamon on each apple half.

4. Stuff the middle with chopped walnuts and sprinkle with honey.

5. Bake for 20 to 25 minutes, or until the apples are soft.

6. Serve warm for a comforting, naturally sweet dessert.

Frozen mango sorbet

Ingredients

- Frozen mango pieces.

- Water or coconut water.

- Honey (Optional)

Instructions

1. Use a food processor or blender to combine frozen mango pieces.

2. Gradually add water or coconut water to the mixture until it has the consistency of sorbet.

3. Optional: Sweeten with honey.

4. Place the sorbet mixture in a container and freeze for at least two hours.

5. Scoop and eat this delightful frozen mango sorbet.

Almond Flour Blueberry Muffins

Ingredients

Ingredients include almond flour, eggs, and baking powder.

- Vanilla Extract

- Blueberries, fresh or frozen.

- Maple syrup.

Instructions

1. Preheat the oven to 350°F/175°C and line a muffin tray with paper liners.

2. In a mixing basin, combine almond flour, eggs, baking powder, vanilla extract, and maple syrup until thoroughly blended.

3. Gently fold in the blueberries.

4. Divide the batter between the muffin cups.

5. Bake for 20-25 minutes, until the muffins are brown and a toothpick inserted comes out clean.

6. Let cool before serving.

Vanilla Chia Seed Pudding With Sliced Almonds

Ingredients

- 1/4 cup chia seeds.

Ingredients: 1 cup almond milk, 1 tablespoon vanilla essence, and sliced almonds.

Instructions

1. In a jar or basin, mix together the chia seeds, almond milk, and vanilla essence.

2. Stir thoroughly and chill for at least 2 hours or overnight.

3. Prior to serving, mix the chia pudding.

4. Layer the chia pudding in serving glasses or bowls.

5. Garnish with sliced almonds for extra crunch.

Lemon Poppy Seed Cake Bites

Ingredients

Ingredients for this recipe include almond flour, lemon zest, poppy seeds, and maple syrup.

- Almond Butter

- Vanilla Extract

Instructions

1. In a bowl, mix almond flour, lemon zest, and poppy seeds.

2. Combine the maple syrup, almond butter, and vanilla essence. Mix until dough forms.

3. Form the dough into bite-size balls.

4. Refrigerate for a minimum of 30 minutes before serving.

Berry and Yogurt Parfait Cones

Ingredients

- Waffle cones with low-fat yogurt.

- Mixed berries, including strawberries, blueberries, and raspberries.

Instructions

1. In a waffle cone, combine low-fat yogurt and mixed berries.

2. Add layers as desired.

3. Serve immediately to create a fun and portable parfait.

Pistachio and Apricot Energy Bites

Ingredients

Chopped dried apricots, pistachios, and almond butter.

- Honey - Rolled oats.

Instructions

1. In a food processor, blend the dried apricots, pistachios, almond butter, honey, and rolled oats.

2. Pulse until the mixture combines.

3. Form the mixture into bite-size energy balls.

4. Refrigerate for a minimum of 30 minutes before serving.

Peach-Mint Sorbet

Ingredients

- Frozen peach slices.

Ingredients: - Fresh mint leaves - Water (or coconut water)

- Honey (Optional)

Instructions

1. Process frozen peach slices, fresh mint leaves, and water or coconut water until smooth.
2. Optional: Sweeten with honey.
3. Place the sorbet mixture in a container and freeze for at least two hours.
4. Scoop and savor this delightful peach and mint sorbet.

Oat Flour Banana Bread

Ingredients

Ingredients: oat flour, mashed ripe bananas, and eggs

Baking soda

Ingredients include cinnamon, vanilla essence, and maple syrup.

Instructions

1. Preheat the oven to 350°F/175°C and oil a loaf pan.
2. In a mixing basin, add oat flour, mashed bananas, eggs, baking soda, cinnamon, vanilla extract, and maple syrup.
3. Mix until well blended.
4. Transfer the batter to the prepared loaf pan.
5. Bake for 45–50 minutes, or until a toothpick inserted comes out clean.
6. Let cool before slicing.

Quinoa Pudding With Raisins

Ingredients

Ingredients include cooked quinoa, almond milk, and raisins.

- Maple syrup.

Ingredients include vanilla extract and cinnamon.

Instructions

1. In a saucepan, boil the almond milk over medium heat.

2. Combine the cooked quinoa, raisins, maple syrup, vanilla essence, and cinnamon.

3. Stir until the mixture thickens and is cooked completely.

4. Serve warm or cold, according to your liking.

Red Raspberry Coconut Chia Popsicles

Ingredients

Ingredients include coconut milk, fresh or frozen raspberries, chia seeds, and maple syrup.

Instructions

1. In a blender, mix the coconut milk, raspberries, chia seeds, and maple syrup.
2. Blend until smooth.
3. Pour the mixture into the popsicle molds.
4. Freeze for at least four hours, or until solid.
5. Run the molds under warm water to remove the popsicles.

Baked Pear with Cinnamon and Honey

Ingredients

Ingredients: - Halved and cored pears - Ground cinnamon.

- Honey

Instructions

1. Preheat your oven to 375°F (190°C).

2. Arrange halved and cored pears on a baking sheet.

3. Sprinkle ground cinnamon on each pear half.

4. Drizzle with honey.

5. Bake for 20–25 minutes, or until the pears are soft.

6. Serve warm as a naturally sweet and warming dessert.

Turmeric Golden Milk Popsicles

Ingredients

- Coconut Milk

- Turmeric Powder

Ingredients include grated ginger and honey.

- Black Pepper

Instructions

1. In a saucepan, heat the coconut milk over medium heat.

2. Combine the turmeric powder, grated ginger, honey, and a sprinkle of black pepper.

3. Stir until thoroughly blended and heated through.

4. Let the mixture cool.

5. Transfer the golden milk mixture to popsicle molds.

6. Freeze for at least four hours, or until solid.

7. Run the molds under warm water to remove the popsicles.

www.ingramcontent.com/pod-product-compliance
Lightning Source LLC
Chambersburg PA
CBHW060956260726
48661CB00005B/1906